Lamiaa Mageed Sayed Ibrahim

Application of Nanotechnology in the Medical Field

Lamiaa Mageed Sayed Ibrahim

Application of Nanotechnology in the Medical Field

Therapeutic Nanomedicine

Scholars' Press

Imprint

Cover image: www.ingimage.com

Publisher:
Scholars' Press
is a trademark of
Dodo Books Indian Ocean Ltd. and OmniScriptum S.R.L publishing group

120 High Road, East Finchley, London, N2 9ED, United Kingdom
Str. Armeneasca 28/1, office 1, Chisinau MD-2012, Republic of Moldova, Europe
Managing Directors: Ieva Konstantinova, Victoria Ursu
info@omniscriptum.com

Printed at: see last page
ISBN: 978-620-9-69565-0

Applications of Nanotechnology in the Medical Field

Therapeutic Nanomedicine

Abstract

Nanotechnology is revolutionizing medicine by enabling highly precise diagnostics, targeted therapies, and personalized healthcare solutions. This review explores the multifaceted applications of nanotechnology across medical fields such as oncology and infectious disease control. Engineered nanoparticles (NPs), such as liposomes, polymeric carriers, and carbon-based nanomaterials, enhance drug solubility, protect therapeutic agents from degradation, and enable site-specific delivery, thereby reducing toxicity to healthy tissues. In diagnostics, nanosensors and contrast agents provide ultra-sensitive detection of biomarkers, supporting early diagnosis and real-time monitoring. Nanotechnology also contributes to regenerative medicine, antimicrobial therapies, wearable devices, and theragnostic, which integrate treatment and diagnosis into unified systems. Advanced innovations such as nanobots and smart nanosystems further extend these capabilities, enabling responsive drug delivery and minimally invasive interventions. Despite its immense potential, nanomedicine faces challenges, including biocompatibility, environmental safety, manufacturing scalability, and regulatory oversight. Addressing these issues is essential for clinical translation and public acceptance. In summary, nanotechnology offers transformative tools that are reshaping medical diagnostics, therapeutics, and disease prevention. Through continued research and interdisciplinary collaboration, it holds the potential to significantly enhance treatment outcomes, reduce healthcare costs, and usher in a new era of precise and personalized medicine.

Keywords: Nanomedicine, Healthcare, Nanoparticles, Clinical applications.

1. Introduction

The term "nanotechnology" is a concept that has only developed in the last decade with the prefix "nano" referred to the Greek word "nanos", representing that something is dwarf-sized. Therefore, the term "nanotechnology" refers to a technology that uses very small particles invisible to the naked eye **[1]**. Before the 19th century, although the term nanotechnology had not yet been globally defined, the applications of nanotechnology were already used in the industrial field **[2]**.

For the first time ever, during a meeting of American Physical Society in 1959, Richard Feynman discussed the term of nanotechnology systematically, laying the foundations of the nanotechnology field **[3]**. Then, at the end of 19th century and early of the 20th century, the field of nanotechnology experienced a massive expansion, when almost all industrialized countries started pursuing nanotechnology research in all fields including medicine **[4]**. Introduction of modern nanotechnology in the medical field aimed at better diagnostics, prevention, and treatment of diseases and was later named "nanomedicine" **(Fig. 1)** **[5]**.

Traditional small molecule drugs have no special selectivity, and they need to pay attention to the frequency and dosage, and can lead to dangerous side effects. They do not pass across some biological barriers, and their efficiency may also affect owing to the poor solubility. In contrast, nanomedicines are targeted and help to enhance bioavailability and reduce drug toxicity. It can slow-release drugs and extend the half-life of them **[6]**. More importantly, the solubility and permeability of insoluble drugs should be improved to make the drugs cross biological barriers **(Fig. 2) [6]**. It is primarily used in disease diagnosis, treatment, monitoring and other drugs or biological products to improve human health **[7, 8]**.

Recently, nanomedicine has great development potential and application prospect in clinical treatment of the tumor. In addition to tumor treatment, it can also be used in anti-infection, ophthalmic disease, neurological disease, gene editing, and immunotherapy. Although nanotechnology has been proposed for decades **[9]**, because of the great changes in physical and chemical properties of nanomaterials, the physicochemical properties and metabolic pathways of nanotechnology still need to be studied **[10]**. There is now broad consensus among medical researchers and practitioners that along with personalized medicine and regenerative medicine, nanomedicine is likely to revolutionize our definitions of what constitutes human disease and its treatment. At present, research on intelligent nanorobots is also very popular. The rise of artificial intelligence (AI) also brings hope for the clinical transformation of nanomedicines **[11]**.

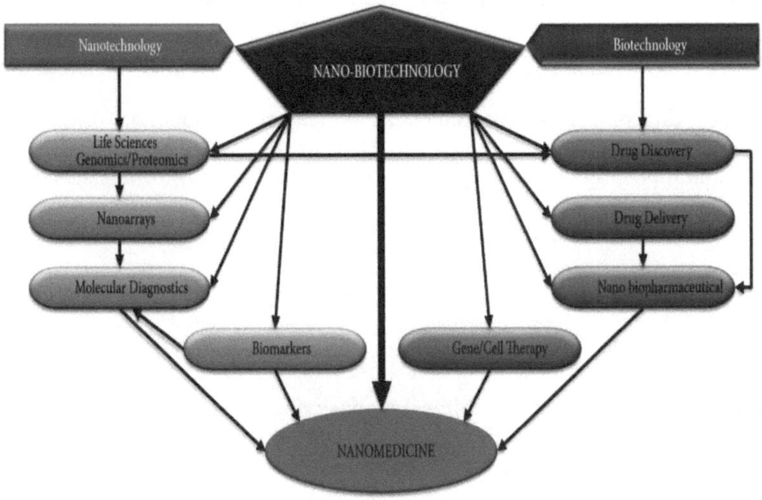

Fig.1: Illustration of how nanomedicine research is based on the application of Nano biotechnology (adapted from **Jain, 2008 [5]**)

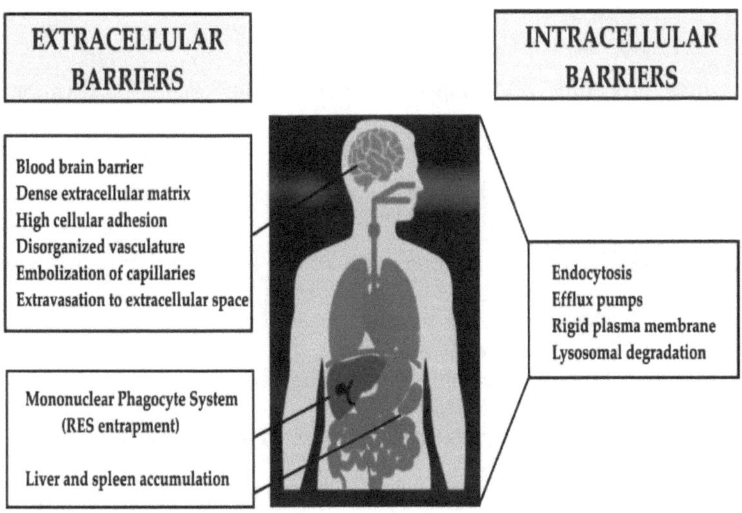

Fig. 2: Biological Barriers [6]

2. Ideal Properties of Nanoparticle Delivery Systems

Nanoparticles are colloidal particles, ranging from 1 to 1000 nm, and are mainly composed of different macromolecules in which the therapeutic drugs can be adsorbed, entrapped, or covalently attached. In the field of drug development, nanoparticles provide significant advantages that can be attributed to their physicochemical properties in order to achieve controlled release characteristics **[12]**. Controlling the product life cycle through reducing dosing frequency creates a potential opportunity that can be achieved by designing nanoparticles with controlled release for drugs that go off-patent. Numerous factors impact the effectiveness of nanoparticles in drug delivery, such as physical and biological stability, good component tolerability, the simplicity of the manufacturing method, ease of manufacturing process scale-up, the convenience of freeze-drying, and sterilization **[12]**.

There are some properties of nanoparticles that are important for drug-delivery application and should be taken into consideration during the development of nanomedicines:

1. It should be characterized by high drug capacity and exhibit a very low possibility of immediate release of the therapeutic agent.

2. It should have the ability to be combined with ligands for targeted drug delivery.

3. It should be stable enough to pass through the biological barriers with respect to their physicochemical properties, such as size, size distribution, surface area, etc.

4. Therapeutic agents should be completely released from nanoparticles at an optimal rate that is based on the formulation design.

5. It should be biocompatible, biodegradable, and non-immunogenic.

6. Organic solvents and toxic ingredients should be excluded from the manufacturing process.

7. All components of the formulation should be safe, affordable and commercially available.

8. Simplicity, affordability, and ease of scaling up are the main characteristics that should be included in the manufacturing process.

9. Nanoparticle formulation should have the ability to be involved in different processes during the manufacturing process, such as lyophilization, sterilization, drying, blending, granulation, compression, capsule filling, and packaging.

10. Nanoparticles should be stable in storage.

3. The Main Types of Nanoparticles Used in Nanomedicines

Nanomedicines contain inorganic nanomaterials (metal & metal oxide nanoparticles, carbon nanotubes, black phosphorus nanoparticles) and organic nanoparticles (dendrimers, polymers, micelles, liposomes, nanocrystals, etc) **(Fig. 3)** **[13]**. Here are some of the more important nanomedicines and their research progress.

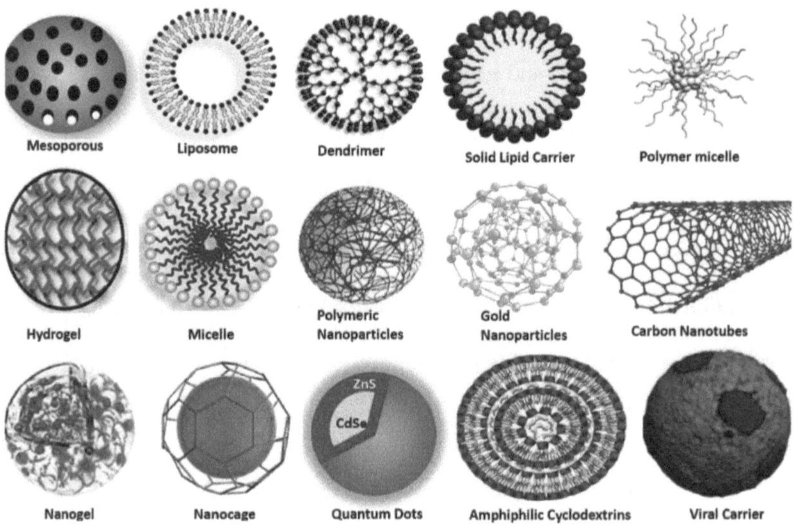

Fig.3: Different types of nanocarriers (nanoparticles) serve as drug delivery in nanomedicines **[13]**

3.1. Nanocrystals

Nanocrystals are colloidal dispersive systems mainly formed by drugs, which can be stabilized and dispersed by modification of a small amount of surfactant or polymer materials **[14]**. They have high drug loading capacity, which approach 100 %. They can improve the solubility and bioavailability of the drugs without carrier materials **[15, 16]**.

3.2. Liposomes

Due to the modifiable sites, liposome nanodrugs have excellent biocompatibility and dependability, which can achieve targeting, improve the water solubility, slow-release drugs, and can also be made into vaccine carriers **[17]**. So far, they are most variety of nanomedicines on the market. The in vivo stability of mesoporous silica nanoparticles can be improved by encapsulating them with liposomes **[18]**. Nevertheless, although the manufacturing process can also reduce their curative effect, liposomes may cause drug leakage when conditions such as the pH or temperature change **[19]**. It has been reported that liposome drugs attracted Immunoglobulin M (IgM) in vivo and induce immunogenicity, and the protein corona of plasma protein formation also affected their targeting **[20]**. Using the apolipoprotein in the plasma as a target factor does not cause immunogenicity, and can be utilized to cross the blood-brain barrier (BBB) **[21]**.

3.3. Black phosphorus (BP)

Carbon nanotubes have recently been added to the SIN ('Substitute It Now') list to their carcinogenicity and reproductive toxicity **[22]**. Though, black phosphorus nanosheets (BPNS) may be used as their new substitution of high drug loading, which has better biocompatibility and rapid degradation **[23, 24]**. In recent years, it has become a research hotspot to study the combination of multiple models and new nanomaterials for the treatment of tumors. BPNS recognize the combination of chemotherapy and photothermal therapy (PTT) for the pulmonary metastatic tumors treatment **[25]**. The combination of photothermal and photodynamic therapy is also indicated, which improves the drug stability **[26]**. Additionally, the newly prepared black phosphorus drugs can also be utilized to assist in the treatment of depression **[27]**. BP has potent biological activity and could be used as an antioxidant in oxidation-reduction targeted therapy, which is a new field to be explored. Hou et al. **[28]** supposed that it could be effectively protected the kidney from reactive oxygen species (ROS) damage by removing ROS in the kidney.

3.4. Gold nanoparticles

Gold nanoparticles (NPs) are made of gold and characterized by safety. Hocevar et al. **[29]** has shown that they do not affect the immune function of B lymphocytes in vitro for the first time. They could be used as materials of photothermal therapy and for the treatment of tumors **[30]**, weight loss therapy and so on **[31, 32]**. The molecular dynamic simulation and experimental photothermal therapy revealed excellent applications of these nanomaterials into nanomedicine for clearing biofilm and stimulating the grown of fibroblast **[33, 34]**. The gold NPs loaded with clustered regularly interspaced short palindromic repeats (CRISPR) can be used to edit the genes of hematopoietic stem cells, promising cures for blood diseases and acquired immune deficiency syndrome (AIDS) **[35]**.

Conversely, gold nanoparticles have the problem of aggregation in vivo which can be prevented through coating gold Nps with protective polymer and making them spherical or selenium (Se-) terminated polyethylene glycol (PEG) and the stability of gold NPs in biological samples can be stimulated **[36]**.

3.5. Polymeric nanomedicines

Polymeric/polymer nanoparticles are materials consisted of polymers, combining metal particles, inorganic nonmetal particles or organic matter at the nanoscale **[37]**. They can be used to treat neurological diseases by improving the drug delivery of the brain, extending the drug blood circulation time and improving the material utilization. Chen et al. **[38]** developed a newly nanodrug for Parkinson's disease, opening up an oral approach that can go through the gastrointestinal and blood-brain barriers.

3.6. Dendrimers

They are special three-dimensional, hyper-branched, globular nanopolymeric structures. They have attractive properities such as water solubility, narrow polydispersity index, nano-scaled size, modifiable molecular structure, internal cavity and numerous peripheral functional groups separate these from other nanosystems. Terminal functionality acts as a platform for the conjugation and targeting of drugs. **[39]**. Dendrimers have been widely examined for biodelivery through transdermal, nasal, ocular, and pulmonary pathways, as well as improving the solubility **[40]**.

3.7. Nanogel

They consisted of of flexible hydrophilic polymers, can be prepared as plain gels. Upon swelling, the drug could be randomly inserted into the nanogel. Consequently, the gel collapses, resulting in the creation of solid, compact nanoparticles with reduced solvent amount. They provide new applications for polymer-based drug carrier systems because of their biocompatibility, high moisture content and suitable mechanical properties **[41]**.

3.8 Quantum dots

Quantum dots (QDs) are considered as semiconductor nanocrystals with a diameter ranging from 2 to 10 nm with their optical characteristics, such as absorbance and photoluminescence being size-dependent **[42]**. The significant interest of QDs have established in the field of nanomedicine, because, unlike traditional organic dyes, QDs pose emissions in the near-infrared region ($<$ 650 nm), a very useful phenomenon in the biomedical imaging field, due to low tissue absorption and decreased light dispersion **[43]**.

4. Clinical Applications of Nanomedicines in Diseases

4.1. Cancer treatment

Nanomedicines have been extensively used in cancer therapy due to their unique features that can increase drug penetration, prolonging the circulation time, and reduce the accumulation of drugs in non-target tissues. It could be explained as the vascular endothelial cell gap of the tumor is large, therefore nanomedicine can enter into the tumor tissue through the vascular endothelial cell gap and enrich, which is called enhanced permeability and retention effect (EPR effect) of the tumor **[44]**. Mitochondria of tumor cells could be utilized as targets for nanomedicine since they produce ROS **[45]**. Increasing the osmotic and promoting cell lysis through nanoparticles containing sodium chloride (NaCl) nanoparticles is also a new way to kill tumors **[46]**. Furthermore, Wang et al. **[47]** suggested the development of nano-gas drugs (that is the gas-releasing nanomedicines), which can be used to release hydrogen (H_2), carbon monoxide (CO), nitric oxide (NO), and hydrogen sulfide (H_2S) to suppress mitochondrial respiration of tumor cells **(Fig. 4) [48]**.

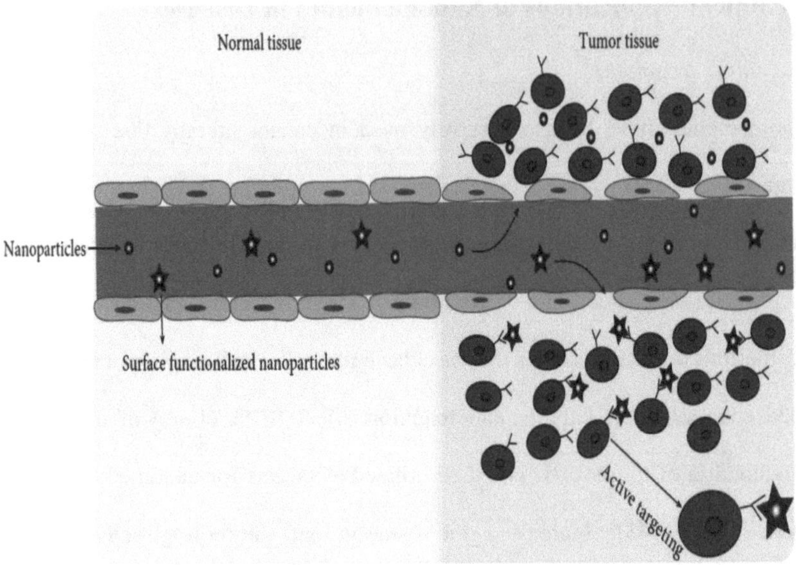

Fig. 4: EPR effect of nanoparticles in tumor tissues and targeting of surface functionalized nanoparticles **[48]**

4.2. Ocular diseases

The antibacterial function and penetrating ability of nanomedicines provide novel ideas for the ocular diseases treatment. Nanomedicines are able to penetrate the physiological ocular barriers, prolong the duration of drug release, extend the residence time of drug molecules in the eye tissue and improve the bioavailability, hence enhancing the therapeutic effect and decreasing the administration frequency **[48]**. Various types of nanomedicines, such as adeno-associated viral (AAV) vectors, liposomes, inorganic nanoparticles, cell-derived derivatives and polymer-drug/protein conjugates, have been developed for the ocular diseases treatment, like diabetic macular edema, inherited retinal disease (IRD), dry eye, glaucoma, and age-related macular degeneration **[49]**.

4.3. Infectious diseases

Nanomedicines have also been developed for the treatment of infectious diseases, such as bacterial/fungal infections, viral infections and parasitic diseases **[48]**. Nanomedicines are a viable substitute for antibiotics. Although the mechanism is not clear, studies have revealed that it has a better effect on antibiotic resistant-bacteria. Because of its targeting, it could reduce the effective concentration of drugs as well as improve the effectiveness of existing antibacterial drugs **[50]**. For viral infections, nanomedicines can be designed as antiviral vaccines or as carriers encapsulating antiviral drugs to target the infected cells, which has been used in the treatment and prevention of viral infections, such as severe acute respiratory syndrome coronavirus 2 (SARS-CoV-2), respiratory syncytial virus (RSV), hepatitis C (HCV), Ebola virus, influenza virus and Zika virus infection **[48]**. Nanomedicines could also be used in the treatment of parasitic infections, for instance, malaria **[48]**.

4.4. Diagnosis and treatment of obesity

The benefit of nanomedicines is to improve the drugs bioavailability to reduce the remarkable toxicity of traditional weight-loss drugs. Nanomedicines for the treatment of obesity and related metabolic diseases are principally through early diagnosis, targeted delivery of drugs, controlling appetite by reducing blood lipid concentration, suppressing fat absorption, transforming white adipose tissue (WAT) into brown-like adipose tissue **[51]**. Using gold nanoparticles can directly eliminate adipose tissue through PTT; it could enhance the uneven liposuction appearance **(Fig. 5) [52]**.

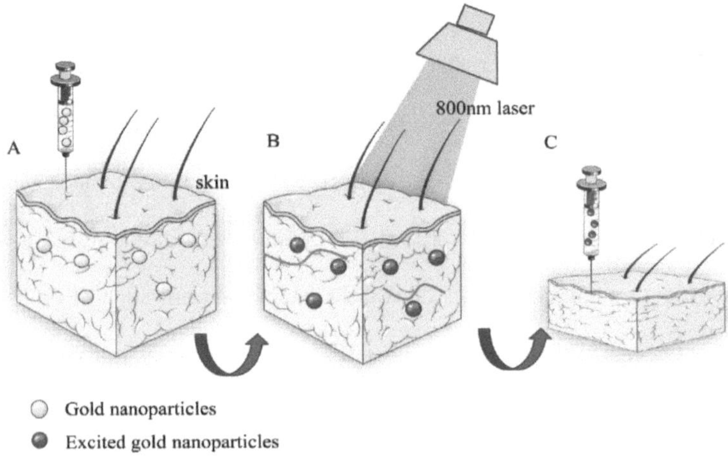

Fig. 5: Treatment of obesity with PTT [52]. (A) Gold nanoparticles are injected into adipose tissue. **(B)** Irradiation of epidermis with 800 nm laser increases the temperature of gold nanoparticles and liquefies small volumes of fat. **(C)** Adipose tissue and gold nanoparticles were removed by a liposuction program.

4.5. Brain diseases

Recently, the nanomedicine used in brain diseases is mostly polymer. For example, Chen et al. **[38]** have developed an orally available drug for Parkinson's disease (PD), which can penetrate the gastrointestinal barrier and blood brain barrier. Nanodrugs could be utilized in mesenchymal stem cells (MSCs) - based therapy that can improve the secretion level of natural stem cells and cross the BBB. It can be served as the recovery treatment of ischemic stroke (IS) **[52]**.

4.6. Pulmonary diseases

For the of pulmonary diseases treatment, the main obstacle is to make drugs through pulmonary surfactant without damaging **[53]**. In the study of Tian et al. **[54]** the nanomedicine indicated a strong ability to go through the pulmonary surfactant film without lung structure damaging. Also, a new nanomedicine offers the opportunity to improve the efficiency of influenza virus vaccines.

4.7. Herat diseases

Prevention and therapy of atherosclerosis can be achieved via suppressing macrophage cell proliferation with nanodrugs loaded with simvastatin, so achieving anti-inflammatory effects and halting the atherosclerosis progression **[48]**. Further, increasing the expression of silent information regulator 1 (SIRT1) in plaque could diagnose atherosclerosis and inhibit its growth **[54]**. Nanomedicines can prevent the side effects of vascular restenosis and thrombosis caused by surgery (such as stent implantation). For example, an atherosclerotic drug, rapamycin (MTOR), could be wrapped in a modified red blood cell membrane and injected into the blood to transport the drug to the plaque without surgery **[48]**.

4.8. Skin diseases

Nanomedicines have been represented for the skin diseases treatment such as acne vulgaris, burns and dermatitis, because of to the ability of penetrating the skin barrier, selectively acting on the target site, or extending the drug residence in the skin **[48]**. For example, Acticoat, a silver nanocrystal-coated polyethylene net for burns treatment, can release silver ions to kill microbes by blocking the cell respiration pathway, interfering with microbial electron transport system components, and producing DNA damage **[55]**.

4.9. Immunological diseases and inflammation

Immunological diseases are mostly caused due to the abnormal functioning of the immune system, which includes rheumatoid arthritis, asthma, multiple sclerosis (MS), systemic lupus erythematosus, inflammatory bowel disease, type-1 diabetes mellitus, and so on. Currently, liposomes, polymer nanoparticles and PEG-drug conjugates have been approved for the treatment of immune diseases, such as Joyclu (2021), Relieva (2019), Zilretta (2017), and Paigebin (2016). Nanotechnology is effective to achieve a slow release pattern and prolong the half-life of the encapsulated drugs, which meets the treatment demands of the immune-related diseases **[48]**.

5. Considerations in Nanomedicine Development

5.1. Chemistry, Manufacturing, and Controls (CMC) considerations

Nanomedicines are more complex than conventional drugs, as they face CMC challenges throughout the development of the product and in the later stage of manufacturing scale-up. Consequently, the first step in developing nanomedicine is to detect practicability through understanding the construction the early formulation to demonstrate the principle in the research. This will confirm that the formulation can reproduce through confirmatory studies, as well as ensure its future safety and efficiency in clinical trials **[12]**. Analytical techniques like nuclear magnetic resonance (NMR), mass spectrometry (MS), chromatography, must be used to recognize the chemical structure of each component involved in nanoparticle formulation **[12]**. The physicochemical features of the early formulated example; i.e., particle size, pH, viscosity, and purity, also required to be identified. The biological properties of nanoparticles are needed to be examined to provide appropriate levels of confidence **[12]**.

5.2. Economic considerations

The total investment required funding the development and scaling-up of nanomedicine manufacture needs to be determined. The overall risk of CMC development will need to be factored into the investment profiles required for analyzing potential nanomedicine programs against other development portfolios. Instruments, manufacturing equipment, and other facilities may be costed for some companies, so these facilities need to be provided in the investment strategies of nanomedicine production aligned with clinical supplies **[12]**.

5.3. Regulatory considerations

Early the Food and Drug Administration (FDA) consultations concerning nanomedicine development will assist in understanding the scientific and regulatory issues related to the product, and in addressing questions regarding the safety, effectiveness, public health impact, and regulatory status **[12]**. For that reason, the development of nanomedicine should follow the usual pathways and processes of drug production with an appropriate evaluation framework. In Europe, the European Medicines Agency (EMA) has established an Expert Working Group, and has released some papers for certain nanomedicines to provide guidance to developers in the preparation of marketing approval applications **[56]**.

6. Developmental Nanomedicines

Pharmaceutical nanomedicine products are presented to play a major role in the universal pharmaceutical market and healthcare. Since 1995, about 70 nanomedicine products have been approved by the FDA and the EMA for marketing and double this number are available in clinical trials **[12]**. Many reports show that the number of medications depends on nanotechnology is growing annually. Every year, new nanomedicines of previously approved drugs enter clinical trials to investigate their improvements with respect to efficiency as compared to conventional formulations **[57]**. This is owing to the rapid growth in research and development (R&D) and the high market demand, which displays the nanotechnology importance in the field of drug delivery. However, the majority of nanomedicines approved to date have revealed a reduced toxicity rather than improved efficacy **[12]**. A diversity of nanoparticle-based drugs has entered the market and is used daily by many patients **(Fig. 6)**. Although anticancer nanomedicines are more currently available than any other drug classes on the market, many formulations are also being advertised for further indications, metabolic disorders, containing autoimmune, ophthalmic conditions, neurological diseases, inflammatory diseases, hematological disorders and others **[57]**. These products are from several companies worldwide, and indicate the nanomedicines success as therapeutic agents **[12]**.

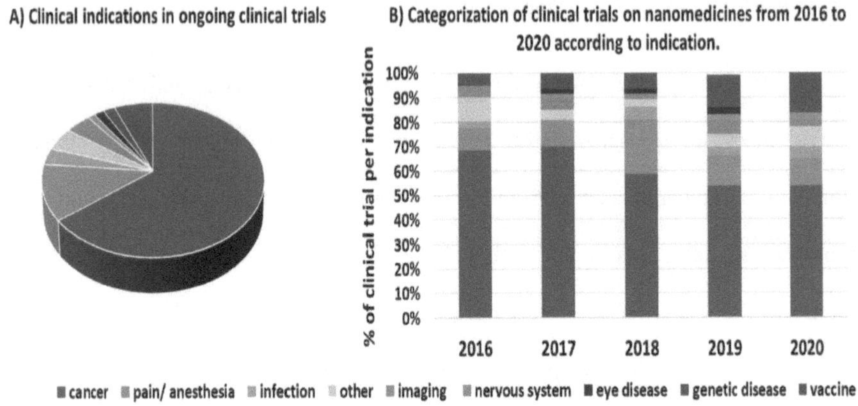

Fig. 6: Categorization of clinical trials based on nanomedicine formulation per indication: A) analysis on all the 409 trials and **B)** repartition per year in the 2016-May 2020 period (333 trials). The analysis was performed on 409 clinical trials identified in the **clinicaltrials.gov** database in May 2020.

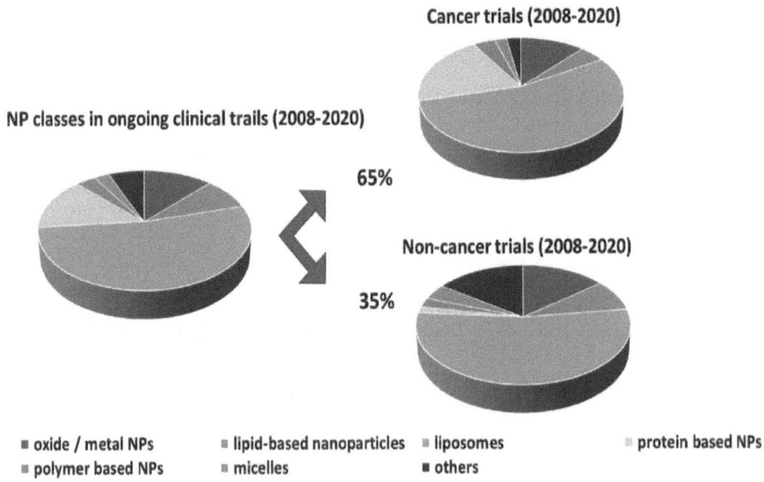

Fig. 7: Nanoparticle classes investigated in ongoing clinical trials. The analysis was performed on 409 clinical trials from 2008 to 2020 identified in the **clinicaltrials.gov** database in May 2020.

7. Potential Reasons for the Failure of Some Nanomedicines

Although the pharmaceutical companies that produce nanomedicines obtain funding from capital markets, and partnerships with industries, clinical failure of some nanomedicine products may arise and cause product terminations or discontinuation and business liquidation **[58]**.

Several nanomedicines act by direct interaction with genetic materials, or by interaction with biomolecules that are required for normal genome function and cell division, all of which can cause genotoxicity and mutagenicity **[59]**. Such toxicity to nanomedicines is mediated by the inflammatory response of neutrophils and macrophages by reactive oxygen and nitrogen species production which result in oxidative and nitrosative stress **[60]**. The free radicals accumulation can lead to extensive damage to the body; including oxidative DNA damage leading to strand breakage, protein denaturation and lipid peroxidation causing cancer, causing damage to mitochondrial membranes leading to cell death and necrosis **[59]**. When administered intravenously, there is a lot of data which indicates nanomedicines accumulation within the liver, and translocation to areas as the central nervous, cardiovascular and renal systems **(Fig. 8)** **[59]**.

At present, the precise interactions of some nanomedicines with biological systems is not yet fully understood, so making understanding, recognizing or drawing conclusions about the physicochemical and toxicological characteristics of nanomedicines difficult **[12]**. Guidance is serious as without it, manufacturers, healthcare providers, the public and policymakers have no clarity and legal certainty. The US FDA, Environmental Protection Agency (EPA), and Health and Consumer Protection Directorate of the European Commission have taken initiatives to deal with the potential risks posed by these nanomedicines **[59]**.

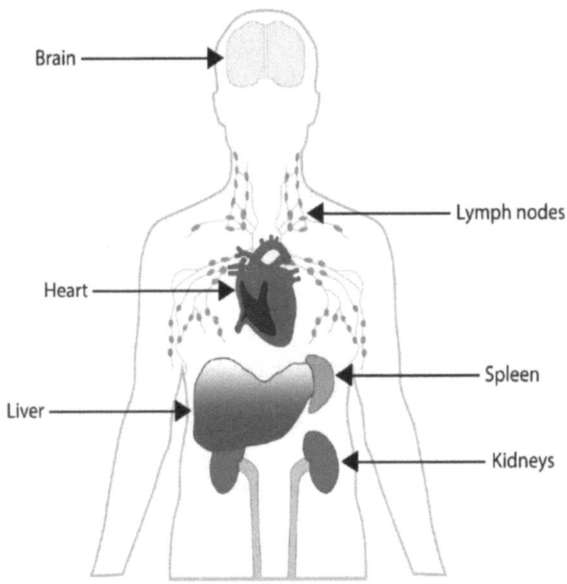

Fig. 8: Schematic representation of the main areas of nanoparticle translocation and accumulation after administration.

8. Challenges and limitations

Despite its remarkable progress, nanomedicine faces a range of scientific, technical, regulatory, and economic challenges that hinder its full clinical integration **(Fig. 9)**. These limitations need to be systematically addressed to realize the field's long-term potential and ensure safe, equitable access to nano-enabled therapies. The barriers to the regulatory systems of various countries are compared to identify the multifaceted challenges associated with ensuring the safety and efficacy of nanomedicine interventions. The lack of consensus not only impedes the research and development (R&D) efforts in nanoparticle-based therapies but also affects the future adoption of nanomedicines. There is an urgent need to establish and implement a coherent and globally synchronized regulatory framework to facilitate the innovation and advancements of nanomedicines.

Addressing these requires collaborative efforts in creating standardized toxicity assays, developing better in vitro/in vivo models, and integrating AI for predictive modeling of nanoparticle behavior.

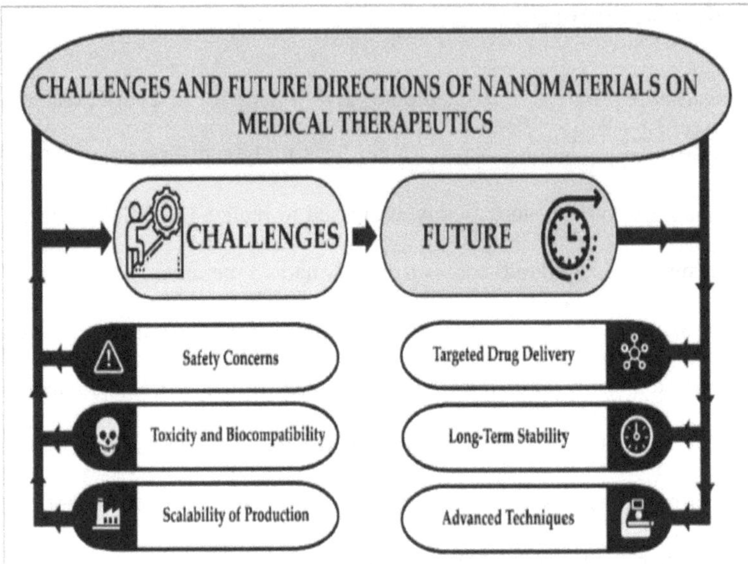

Fig. 9: Challenges and future directions of NMs on medical therapeutics

9. Conclusions and Future Prospects

Nanotechnology is already starting to have an impact on the healthcare system, as various nanotechnology ideas have been developed, and numerous nanotechnology-based medicines are now on the market. Extending the evolution and interest in the nanotechnology field from the last two decades is predicted for future positive progresses in nanomedicines. Therefore, the future of nanomedicines is likely to follow two paths. The first path has been already determined, where nanomedicines are mostly and still developed for cancer indications; as most available nanomedicines in the market are anticancer. The second one is developing nanomedicines to target various diseases other than cancers. Further developments along the second path may be needed to increase the nanomedicines applications to those diseases that cannot be effectively addressed with Conventional drug delivery systems (CDDSs). For instance, nanomedicine in medical diagnosis will permit detection and investigation of tissues in more details: at the cellular and molecular levels, using particular devices **[12]**. Additionally, to get best benefits from the nanoparticle-based strategy for drug delivery, in vitro and in vivo studies require to be further followed to recognize the behaviors of nanoparticles to accelerate nanomedicines through clinical development, and then provide them to the patients. Furthermore, in 2016, the global market size of nanomedicine reached USD 138.8

billion, and by 2025, it is predicted to reach USD 350.8 billion **(Fig. 10)**. This reveals the significance of nanotechnology in the drug delivery field **[12]**.

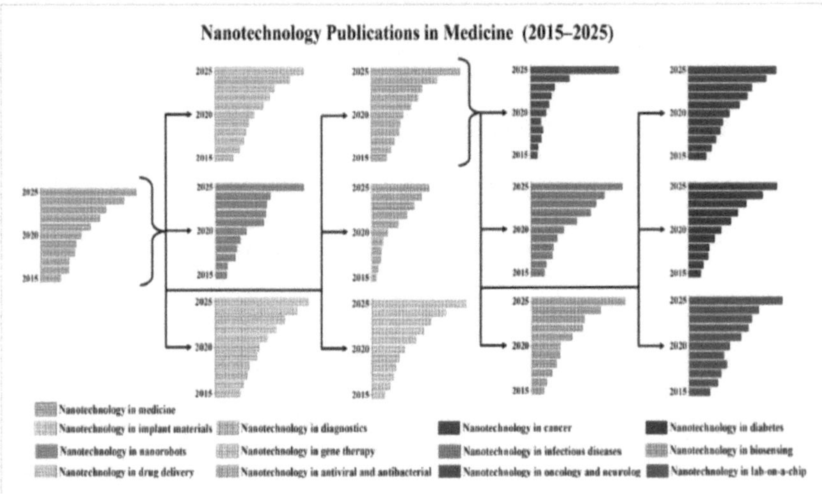

Fig. 10: Annual publication counts in medical nanotechnology (2015-2025). Data source: Scopus; accessed October 2025.

10. Egyptian Experience

In Egypt, several research groups are involved in the development of nanomedicines for advanced drug-delivery applications. This contains the usage of nanocarriers for improving the efficiency of various pharmaceutical productions including oral, nasal, parenteral, pulmonary, transdermal or topical formulations **[61]**. Among the Egyptian laboratories most contributing to the nanomedicine field, Cancer Nanotechnology Research Laboratory (CNRL) established in 2014 at Faculty of Pharmacy, Alexandria University. The number of patients diagnosed with cancer in Egypt increases annually. Therefore, numerous studies concerning the cancer nanomedicine area have been developed by CNRL researchers, particularly for the treatment of lung, breast and liver cancers widely spread in Egypt **[61]**. Another promising research center is the Nanomedicine Division, Center for Materials Science, University of Science and Technology, Zewail City of Science and Technology. Researchers of this group designed novel nanocarriers for different applications including cancer, diabetes and wound healing. Additionally, several research groups have recently focused on the development of nanocarrier formulations for advanced drug-delivery applications in the field of nanomedicine **[61]**.

In 2017, the study of Elzoghby et al. **[62]** affirmed that the superior antitumor efficacy of oral administration of exemestane (EXM) and resveratrol (RES) nanoformulation for breast cancer therapy by increasing their solubility and permeability using hydrophobic proteins. Furthermore, nanoparticles have been widely utilized for topical drug delivery for wound healing. Gold nanoparticles have been used due to their strong antibacterial feature mainly mediated through binding to bacterial DNA and creating holes in cell walls causing cell death. Therefore, gold nanoparticles (28.9–37.65 nm) were embedded in poloxamer/hydroxypropyl methyl cellulose (HPMC) thermoresponsive gels for wound healing purposes to prevent the side effects of antibiotic therapy **[63]**.

In recent years, in the study of El-Sayed et al. **[64]** suggested that incorporation of Au-NPs into *Ficus carica* leaves extract improved its anti-oxidative properties and hence reduced the oxidative toxicity and kidney damage induced by cisplatin. Also, the Au-NPs that was produced perfectly by microwave radiation technique, was evaluated for treating the complications occurred as a result of oxidative stress and their adverse effects at the induced hyperglycemic conditions **[65]**. Consequently, Abu-Taweel et al. **[66]** has been completed the study of nanoparticles against experimentally induced diabetes and found that curcumin nanoparticles exhibited an effective role in regulating levels of glucose and insulin, improving oxidative stability, restoring tetrahydrobiopterin (BH4) levels and improving the bioavailability of nitric oxide (NO) in the vascular walls.

In addition, the study of Salma et al. **[67]** indicated that titanium dioxide nanoparticles (TiO_2 NPs) have the potential to be used in nanomedicine for cancer diagnosis and therapy owing to their valuable properties such as biocompatibility, photocatalytic activity and good optical and electronic characteristics. Therefore, it is suggested to study and explore the medical, biological and toxicological effects of TiO_2 NPs. Recently, NPs might be conjugated with proteins and immunoglobulins

(IgGs) that could assist in specific diagnosis of many parasitic diseases, like Malaria, Toxoplasmosis and Amebiasis, besides, reduced harmful side effects and improved efficiency can be provided by immobilizing antiparasitic medicines on or inside nanomaterials **[68]**.

Moreover, Mazayen et al. **[69]** displayed the vital role of nanotechnology in the nanomedicine development of therapeutic formulations for the diagnosis, progress and treatment of long-term human immunity against COVID-19 and the importance of nanoparticles in vaccination against COVID-19.

References

1. **Rabie A, Abd-Ellah O, Abuelwafa E, et al**. Nanotechnology and Nanomedicine-Based Strategies in Parasitic Infection [A Review Article]. Egyptian Journal of Veterinary Sciences, 2025: 1-9. doi: 10.21608/ejvs.2025.425198.3135

2. **Anup Basnet C**. Nanomedicine In 2025: Current Trends and Future Prospects. J Recent Adv Nanomed & Nanotech. 2025; 1(3): 555570.

3. **Colman D**. Richard Feynman introduces the world to nanotechnology with two seminal lectures (1959 & 1984). 2013. Open Culture (openculture.com).

4. **Chan C**. From nanotech to nanoscience. 2008. Distillations. Science History Institute.

5. **Jain KK**. Nanomedicine: application of nanobiotechnology in medical practice. 2008. Medical Principles and Practice. 17(2): 89–101.

6. **Wang X, Ho C, Tsatskis Y, et al**. Intracellular manipulation and measurement with multipole magnetic tweezers. 2019. Sci. Robot. 4 (28): eaav6180.

7. **Jeong U, Herricks T, Shahar E, et al**. Amorphous Se: a new platform for synthesizing superparamagnetic colloids with controllable surfaces. 2005. J. Am. Chem. Soc. 127 (4): 1098–1099.

8. **Kaehler T**. Nanotechnology: basic concepts and definitions. 1994. Clin. Chem. 40 (9): 1797–1799.

9. **Shao S, Zhou Q, Si J, et al**. A non-cytotoxic dendrimer with innate and potent anticancer and anti-metastatic activities. 2017. Nat. Biomed. Eng. 1 (9): 745–757.

10. **Singh AV, Ansari P, Laux A**. Micro-nanorobots: important considerations when developing novel drug delivery platforms. 2019. Expert Opin. Drug Deliv. 16 (11): 1259–1275.

11. **Li Y, Lu H, Liang S, et al**. Dual stable nanomedicines prepared by cisplatin-crosslinked camptothecin prodrug micelles for effective drug delivery. 2019. ACS Appl. Mater. Interfaces 11 (23): 20649–20659.

12. **Halwani AA**. Development of pharmaceutical nanomedicines: from the bench to the market. 2022. Pharmaceutics. 14(106): 1-21.

https://doi.org/10.3390/ pharmaceutics14010106

13. **Yaqoob AA, Ahmad H, Parveen T, et al**. Recent advances in metal decorated nanomaterials and their various biological applications: A Review. 2020. Front. Chem. 8:341.

doi: 10.3389/fchem.2020.00341

14. **Liu B, Deng X, Xie Z, et al**. Thiol-Ene click reaction as a facile and general approach for surface functionalization of colloidal nanocrystals. 2017. Adv. Mater. (Deerfield Beach, Fla.) 29 (36): 1604878 (1-9).

15. **Chai Z, Ran D, Lu L, et al**. Ligand-modified cell membrane enables the targeted delivery of drug nanocrystals to glioma. 2019. ACS Nano. 13 (5):5591–5601.

16. **Wang Y, Zhang K, Qin X, et al**. Biomimetic nanotherapies: red blood cell-based core-shell structured nanocomplexes for atherosclerosis management. 2019. Adv. Sci. (Weinh) 6 (12): 1900172.

17. **Wang J, Li P, Yu Y, et al**. Pulmonary surfactant–biomimetic nanoparticles potentiate heterosubtypic influenza immunity. 2020. Science. 367 (6480): eaau0810.

18. **Durfee PN, Lin YS, Dunphy DR, et al**. Mesoporous silica nanoparticle-supported lipid bilayers (Protocells) for active targeting and delivery to individual leukemia cells. 2016. ACS Nano. 10 (9): 8325–8345.

19. **Ghasemiyeh P and Mohammadi-Samani S**. Solid lipid nanoparticles and nanostructured lipid carriers as novel drug delivery systems: applications, advantages and disadvantages. 2018. Res. Pharm. Sci. 13 (4): 288–303.

20. **Monopoli MP, Aberg C, Salvati A, et al**. Biomolecular coronas provide the biological identity of nanosized materials. 2012. Nat. Nanotechnol. 7 (12): 779–786.

21. **Zhang Z, Guan J, Jiang Z, et al**. Brain-targeted drug delivery by manipulating protein corona functions. 2019. Nat. Commun. 10 (1): 3561.

22. **Hansen SF and Lennquist A**. Carbon nanotubes added to the SIN List as a nanomaterial of very High Concern. 2020. Nat. Nanotechnol. 15 (1): 3–4.

23. **Yang X, Wang D, Zhu J, et al**. Functional black phosphorus nanosheets for mitochondria-targeting photothermal/photodynamic synergistic cancer therapy. 2019. Chem. Sci. 10 (13): 3779–3785.

24. **Wang H, Yang X, Shao W, et al**. Ultrathin black phosphorus nanosheets for efficient singlet oxygen generation. 2015. J. Am. Chem. Soc. 137 (35): 11376–11382.

25. **Hu K, Xie L, Zhang Y, et al**. Marriage of black phosphorus and $Cu^{(2+)}$ as effective photothermal agents for PET-guided combination cancer therapy. 2020. Nat. Commun. 11 (1): 2778.

26. **Wang S, Shao J, Li Z, et al**. Black phosphorus-based multimodal nanoagent: showing targeted combinatory therapeutics against cancer metastasis. 2019. Nano Lett. 19 (8): 5587–5594.

27. **Jin L, Hu P, Wang Y, et al**. Fast-acting black-phosphorus-assisted depression therapy with low toxicity. 2020. Adv. Mater. 32 (2): e1906050.

28. **Hou J, Wang H, Ge Z, et al**. Treating acute kidney injury with antioxidative black phosphorus nanosheets. 2020. Nano Lett. 20 (2): 1447–1454.

29. **Hocevar S, Milosevic A, Rodriguez-Lorenzo L, et al**. Polymer-coated gold nanospheres do not impair the innate immune function of human B lymphocytes in vitro. 2019. ACS Nano 13 (6): 6790–6800.

30. **Singh AV, Jahnke T, Kishore V, et al**. Cancer cells biomineralize ionic gold into nanoparticles-microplates via secreting defense proteins with specific gold-binding peptides. 2018. Acta Biomater. 71: 61–71.

31. **Benyettou F, Ramdas A, Dho Y, et al**. Aqueous synthesis of triphenylphosphine-modified gold nanoparticles for synergistic in vitro and in vivo photothermal chemotherapy. 2020. Chemistry 26 (23): 5270–5279.

32. **Sheng W, Alhasan A, DiBernardo G, et al**. Gold nanoparticle-assisted selective photothermolysis of adipose tissue (NanoLipo), plastic and reconstructive surgery. 2014. Glob. Open J. 2 (12): e283.

33. **Singh V, Kashyap S, Yadav U, et al**. Nitrogen doped carbon quantum dots demonstrate no toxicity under in vitro conditions in a cervical cell line and in vivo in Swiss albino mice. 2019. Toxicol. Res. (Camb) 8 (3): 395–406.

34. **Singh A, Jahnke T, Xiao Y, et al**. Peptide-induced biomineralization of tin oxide (SnO(2)) nanoparticles for antibacterial applications. 2019. J. Nanosci. Nanotechnol. 19 (9): 5674–5686.

35. **Shahbazi R, Sghia-Hughes G, Reid J, et al**. Targeted homology-directed repair in blood stem and progenitor cells with CRISPR nanoformulations. 2019. Nat. Mater. 18 (10): 1124–1132.

36. **Xue Y, Dong B, Liu X, et al**. Using selenium-conjugated polyethylene glycol to enhance the stability of gold nanoparticles in biologically relevant samples. 2019. Sci. China-Chem. 62: 280–286.

37. **Liu S, Wang L, Lin M, et al**. Tumor photothermal therapy employing photothermal inorganic nanoparticles/polymers nanocomposites. 2019. Chin. J. Polym. Sci. 37 (2): 115–128.

38. **Chen T, Liu W, Xiong S, et al**. Nanoparticles mediating the sustained Puerarin release facilitate improved brain delivery to treat Parkinson's disease. 2019. ACS Appl. Mater. Interfaces 11 (48) 45276–45289.

39. **Manikkath J, Hegde AR, Kalthur G, et al**. Influence of peptide dendrimers and sonophoresis on the transdermal delivery of ketoprofen. 2017. International Journal of Pharmaceutics 521(1-2): 110-119.

40. **Gothwal A, Malik S, Gupta U, et al**. Toxicity and biocompatibility aspects of dendrimers. 2020. Pharmaceutical Applications of Dendrimers, 251-274. https://doi.org/10.1016/B978-0-12-814527-2.00011-1

41. **Soni G and Yadav KS**. Nanogels as potential nanomedicine carrier for treatment of cancer: A mini review of the state of the art. 2016. Saudi Pharmaceutical Journal 24(2): 133-139.

42. **Pathak G, Hegde G and Prasad V**. Octadecylamine-capped CdSe/ZnS quantum dot dispersed cholesteric liquid crystal for potential display application: Investigation on photoluminescence and UV absorbance. 2020. Liquid Crystals 1-9.

43. **Drissi LB, Ouarrad H, Ramadan FZ, et al**. Graphene and silicene quantum dots for nanomedical diagnostics. 2020. RSC Advances 10(2): 801-811.

44. **Sun B, Luo C, Zhang X, et al**. Probing the impact of sulfur/selenium/carbon linkages on prodrug nanoassemblies for cancer therapy. 2019. Nat. Commun. 10 (1): 3211.

45. **Tian Z, Xu L, Chen Q, et al**. Treatment of surgical brain injury by immune tolerance induced by peripheral intravenous injection of biotargeting nanoparticles loaded with brain antigens. 2019. Front. Immunol. 10: 743.

46. **Jiang W, Yin L, Chen H, et al**. NaCl nanoparticles as a cancer therapeutic. 2019. Adv. Mater. 31 (46): e1904058.

47. **Wang Y, Yang T and He Q**. Strategies for engineering advanced nanomedicines for gas therapy of cancer. 2020. Sci. Rev. 7 (9): 1485–1512.

48. **Li Z, Zhao T, Li J, et al**. Nanomedicine based on natural products: improving clinical application potential. 2022. Journal of Nanomaterials 2022 (1-11) Article ID 3066613. https://doi.org/10.1155/2022/3066613

49. **Srinivasarao DA, Lohiya G and Katti DS**. Fundamentals, challenges and nanomedicine-based solutions for ocular diseases. 2019. Wiley Interdiscip Rev Nanomed Nanobiotechnol 11:e1548.

50. **Jelinkova P, Mazumdar A, Sur VP, et al**. Nanoparticle-drug conjugates treating bacterial infections. 2019. J. Control. Release 307: 166–185.

51. **Wu Z, Chen C, Zhang B, et al**. EGFP-EGF1-conjugated poly(lactic-co-glycolic acid) nanoparticles, a new diagnostic tool and drug carrier for atherosclerosis. 2019. Int. J. Nanomed. 14: 2609–2618.

52. **Sheng W, Seare WJ, DiBernardo B, et al.** A single-blind study evaluating the efficacy of gold nanoparticle photothermal-assisted liposuction in an ex vivo human tissue model. 2018. Aesthet. Surg. J. 38 (11): 1213–1224.

53. **Zhang T, Li F, Xu Q, et al.** Ferrimagnetic nanochains-based mesenchymal stem cell engineering for highly efficient post-stroke recovery. 2019. Adv. Funct. Mater. 29 (24): 1900603.

54. **Lamb YN**. Inclisiran: first approval. 2021. Drugs 81:389-95.

55. **Hashmi DL and Haith L**. The current state of topical burn treatments: a review. 2019. Curr Trauma Rep. 5:160-168.

56. **Soares S, Sousa J, Pais A, et al.** Nanomedicine: principles, properties, and regulatory issues. 2018. Front. Chem. 6: 360. doi: 10.3389/fchem.2018.00360

57. **Farjadian F, Ghasemi A, Gohari O, et a**l. Nanopharmaceuticals and nanomedicines currently on the market: Challenges and opportunities. 2019. Nanomedicine 14: 93–126.

58. **He H, Liu L, Morin E, et al.** Survey of Clinical Translation of Cancer Nanomedicines-Lessons Learned from Successes and Failures. 2019. Acc. Chem. Res. 52: 2445–2461.

59. **Foulkes R, Man E, Thind J, et al.** The regulation of nanomaterials and nanomedicines for clinical application: current and future perspectives. 2020. Biomater. Sci. 8: 4653–4664.

60. **Smolkova B, Dusinska M and Gabelova A**. Nanomedicine and epigenome. Possible health risks. 2017. Food Chem. Toxicol. 109: 780–796.

61. **Elzoghby AO**. Pharmaceutical nanotechnology in Egypt: diverse applications and promising outcomes. 2019. Nanomedicine (Lond.) 14(6): 649–653.

62. **Elzoghby AO, El-Lakany SA, Helmy MW, et al**. Shell-crosslinked zein nanocapsules for oral codelivery of exemestane and resveratrol in breast cancer therapy. 2017. Nanomedicine 12(24): 2785–2805.

63. **Arafa MG, El-Kased RF and Elmazar M**. Thermoresponsive gels containing gold nanoparticles as smart antibacterial and wound healing agents. 2018. *Sci. Rep.* 8(1): 13674.

64. **El-Sayed SM, El-Naggar ME, Hussein J, et al.** Effect of *Ficus carica* L. leaves extract loaded gold nanoparticles against cisplatin-induced acute kidney injury. Colloids and Surfaces B: 2019. Biointerfaces, 184: 110465.

65. **Hussein J, El-Naggar ME, Fouda MMG, et al.** Eco-friendly Microwave Synthesis of Gold Nanoparticles for Attenuation of Brain Dysfunction in Diabetic Rats. Journal of Cluster Science 2020. doi.org/10.1007/s10876-020-01801-y.

66. **Abu-Taweel GM, Attia MF, Hussein J, et al.** Curcumin nanoparticles have potential antioxidant effect and restore tetrahydrobiopterin levels in experimental diabetes. Biomedicine & Pharmacotherapy 2020. 131: 110688.

67. **Salama B, El-Sherbini ES, El-Sayed G, et al**. Applications of titanium dioxide nanoparticles in nanomedicine. 2021. Mansoura Veterinary Medical Journal 22(3): 111-116.

68. **Elhefny MT, Mostafa NE, Mohamed EA, et al**. Role of Nanoparticles in Diagnosis and Management of Parasitic Diseases: Review Article. 2022. The Egyptian Journal of Hospital Medicine 86: 85-89.

69. **Mazayen ZM, Ghoneim AM, Elbatanony RS, et al**. pharmaceutical nanotechnology: from the bench to the market. 2022. Future Journal of Pharmaceutical Sciences 8:12. https://doi.org/10.1186/s43094-022-00400-0

Table of contents

FSC
www.fsc.org
MIX
Papier | Fördert gute Waldnutzung
FSC® C083411

Kolibri 360 GmbH
Ferdinand-Jühlke-Straße 7
99095 Erfurt, Deutschland
produktsicherheit@kolibri360.de

Druck:
CPI Druckdienstleistungen GmbH
im Auftrag der
Kolibri 360 GmbH
Ferdinand-Jühlke-Str. 7
99095 Erfurt